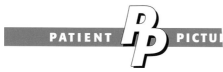

Clinical drawings for your

Urological surgery

Second edition

by Roger S Kirby MA MD FRCS(Urol) FEBU
Consultant Urologist,
St George's Hospital,
London, UK

Series Editor: J Richard Smith MD MRCOG
Consultant Gynaecologist,
Chelsea and Westminster Hospital, London,
and Honorary Senior Lecturer in Obstetrics and Gynaecology,
Imperial College School of Medicine, London, UK

Illustrated by Dee McLean, MeDee Art, London, UK

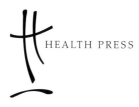

HEALTH PRESS

Oxford

Patient Pictures – Urological surgery
First published 1996
Second edition June 2001

Text © 2001 Roger S Kirby
© 2001 in this edition Health Press Limited
Health Press Limited, Elizabeth House, Queen Street,
Abingdon, Oxford OX14 3JR, UK
Tel: +44 (0)1235 523233
Fax: +44 (0)1235 523238

Patient Pictures is a trade mark of Health Press Limited.

The publisher and author have made every effort to ensure
the accuracy of this book, but cannot accept responsibility
for any errors or omissions.

A CIP catalogue record for this title is available from the
British Library.

ISBN 1-903734-07-X

Printed by Ethedo Press Limited, High Wycombe, Bucks, UK

Reproduction authorization

The purchaser of this *Patient Pictures* series title is hereby authorized to reproduce, by photocopy only, any part of the pictorial and textual material contained in this work for non-profit, educational or patient education use. Photocopying for these purposes only is welcomed and free from further permission requirements from the publisher and free from any fee.

The reproduction of any material from this publication outside the guidelines above is strictly prohibited without the permission in writing of the publisher and is subject to minimum charges laid down by the Publishers Licensing Society Limited or its nominees.

Sarah Redston

Publisher, Health Press Limited, Oxford

Author's preface

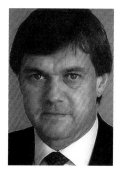

In this 'information' age, it is essential for all doctors to offer patients a full explanation about their diagnosis and recommended treatment. However, even though doctors try their best to provide a clear and simple explanation of the options and what is to happen, the medical jargon they use can be difficult for patients to understand properly. Often, a picture can convey more information than many sentences.

In this book we have tried to illustrate, in a simple manner, the many operations that a urologist has to offer his or her patient. Concise explanations accompany these diagrams, which are designed to answer the questions that patients considering surgery, together with their relatives, are likely to ask. The pictures also provide hard copy that the patient can take home.

In an era when patients are increasingly less disposed to believe unquestioningly that 'doctor knows best', we hope that this book will facilitate the effective two-way communication between physicians and their patients that is so fundamental to good quality care.

Roger S Kirby MA MD FRCS(Urol) FEBU
Consultant Urologist, St George's Hospital, London, UK

The male urinary tract

- The urinary tract is responsible for the production, storage and passing of urine. It includes the kidneys, ureters, bladder and urethra.

- The two kidneys lie at the back of the abdomen. They produce urine by 'filtering' unwanted substances from the blood. The urine produced passes out of the kidneys, down both ureters and into the bladder, where it is stored.

- The bladder fills with urine over 3–4 hours. As it fills, you become increasingly aware of the need to pass urine. During urination, urine passes from the bladder down the urethra to the outside. This involves simultaneous relaxation of the muscles of the urethra and contraction of the muscle of the bladder.

- In men, the urinary and genital tracts overlap. Semen is made in the testes (testicles) and passed up two tubes (called the vas deferens) to be stored in the seminal vesicles behind the prostate. At ejaculation, the bladder neck closes and semen passes down the urethra and out through the penis.

- The prostate is a small gland just below the bladder that fits around the urethra rather like a collar. The prostate produces a fluid that forms part of the semen.

- In men over 40, the prostate often enlarges gradually and presses on the urethra causing obstruction. This can make it difficult to pass urine and you may be unable to empty your bladder completely. You may also feel the need to pass urine more often and more urgently.

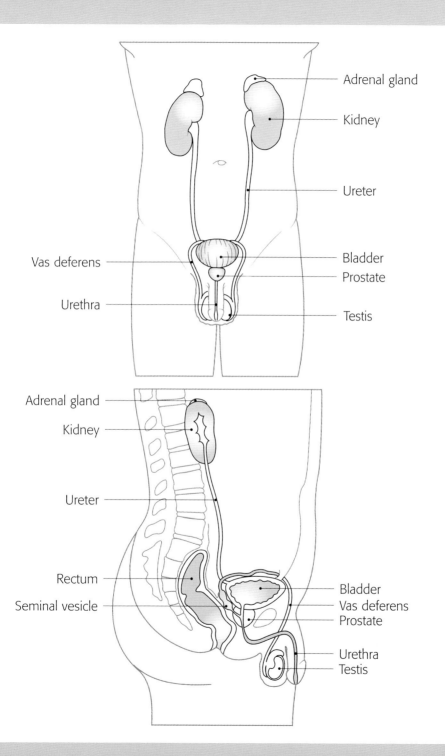

Adrenal gland

Kidney

Ureter

Bladder
Prostate

Testis

Vas deferens

Urethra

Adrenal gland
Kidney

Ureter

Rectum
Seminal vesicle

Bladder
Vas deferens
Prostate

Urethra
Testis

The female urinary tract

- The urinary tract is responsible for the production, storage and passing of urine. It includes the kidneys, ureters, bladder and urethra.

- The two kidneys lie at the back of the abdomen. They produce urine by 'filtering' unwanted substances from the blood. The urine produced passes out of the kidneys, down both ureters and into the bladder, where it is stored.

- The bladder fills with urine over 3–4 hours. As it fills, you become increasingly aware of the need to pass urine. During urination, urine passes from the bladder down the urethra to the outside. This involves simultaneous relaxation of the muscles of the urethra and contraction of the muscle of the bladder.

- Women are more likely to suffer from urinary tract infections (UTIs) than men because the female urethra is much shorter. Emptying your bladder shortly after sex may help to avoid UTIs.

- After childbirth, many women leak small amounts of urine when they cough or sneeze. This is called 'stress incontinence' and occurs when the pelvic floor muscles have been weakened by the passage of the baby down the birth canal. Performing pelvic floor exercises may help strengthen the muscles and stop urine leaking out.

- The flow of urine may be obstructed if the urethra is narrowed by scar tissue or the muscles of the urethra fail to relax. However, this is uncommon.

2

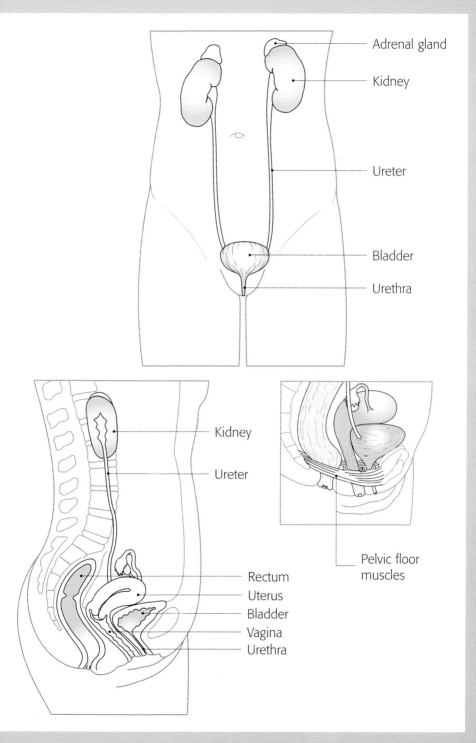

Adrenal gland

Kidney

Ureter

Bladder

Urethra

Kidney

Ureter

Pelvic floor
muscles

Rectum
Uterus
Bladder
Vagina
Urethra

© Health Press Limited

Nephrectomy

- Radical nephrectomy is an operation used to treat kidney cancer that has not spread to the lymph nodes, lungs or bones. It involves removing the entire kidney and often the adrenal gland, as well as the surrounding fat and lymph glands on the affected side.

- The operation is performed under a general anaesthetic and takes about 2 hours.

- During the operation, a catheter is passed up the urethra into the bladder to measure the amount of urine being produced by the remaining healthy kidney. This tube will be removed after 2–3 days.

- After the operation, you may feel some discomfort in your side, particularly when you move or cough, but this can be controlled with painkillers.

- The average hospital stay is 7–10 days, but complete recovery usually takes another 6 weeks.

- If the cancer is removed completely, no further treatment will be required. However, you will need to visit the clinic every 3–6 months for at least 5 years and occasionally have a chest X-ray to check that the cancer has not recurred in your lungs.

- If the cancer is small, an operation called a partial nephrectomy may be performed. Only the portion containing the cancer is removed leaving most of the kidney in place.

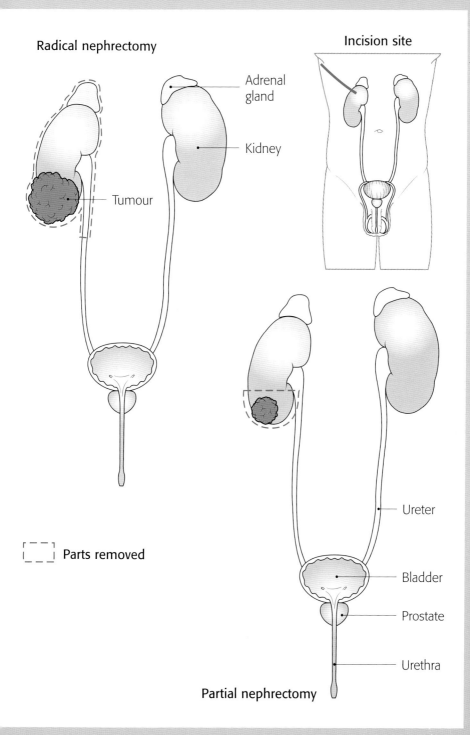

Radical nephrectomy

Incision site

Adrenal gland

Kidney

Tumour

Parts removed

Partial nephrectomy

Ureter

Bladder

Prostate

Urethra

Pyeloplasty

- If the junction where the pelvis of the kidney and ureter meet is narrowed, urine will not drain properly out of the kidney, through the renal pelvis and into the ureter. This is called pelviureteric junction (PUJ) obstruction and you will need an operation called a pyeloplasty.

- The operation involves reconstructing the narrowed area around a small tube called a stent. After 7–10 days, the stent will be removed by cutting the stitch and pulling the tube out.

- The operation is performed under a general anaesthetic and takes 1–2 hours.

- During the operation, a catheter is passed up the urethra into the bladder. This will be removed after a few days. After the operation, you may feel some discomfort in your side but this can be controlled with painkillers.

- The average hospital stay is 7–10 days and complete recovery takes about 3 months. You will need to visit the clinic again once or twice for more X-rays and scans to check that the operation has been a success.

- Occasionally, scar tissue can form and obstruct the flow of urine again. If this happens, you may need to have a further procedure to relieve the obstruction.

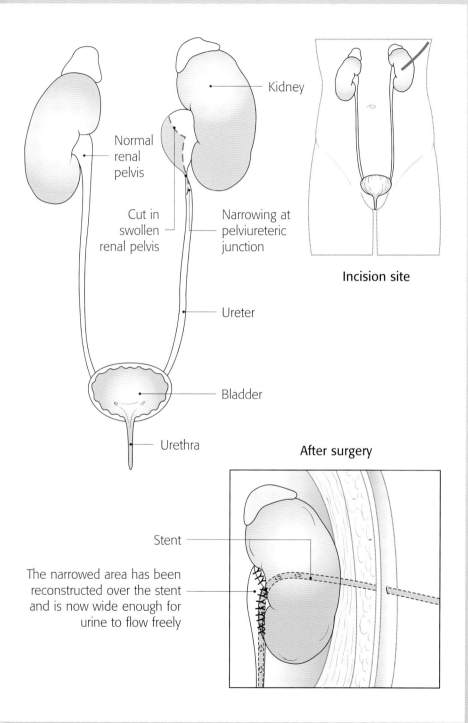

Kidney

Normal renal pelvis

Cut in swollen renal pelvis

Narrowing at pelviureteric junction

Incision site

Ureter

Bladder

Urethra

After surgery

Stent

The narrowed area has been reconstructed over the stent and is now wide enough for urine to flow freely

Nephro-ureterectomy

- Nephro-ureterectomy is an operation to treat cancer affecting the renal pelvis or ureter which drain urine from the kidney.

- The operation involves removing the entire kidney, adrenal gland, ureter and surrounding fat on the affected side. This usually requires two incisions.

- During the operation, a catheter is passed up the urethra into the bladder and a drainage tube is inserted into the wound. The catheter and drainage tube are usually removed after 3–4 days. After the operation, you may feel some discomfort but this can be controlled with painkillers.

- The average hospital stay is 7–10 days and complete recovery takes at least 2–3 months.

- Because these cancers develop from the lining of the urinary tract, they may recur either in the bladder or in the other kidney or ureter. For this reason, you will need to visit the clinic for annual X-rays of the kidney and 3–6-monthly examinations of the bladder (cystoscopy).

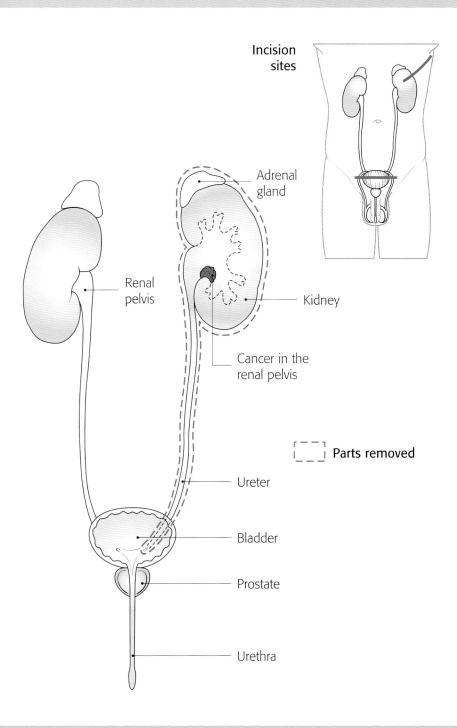

Incision
sites

Adrenal
gland

Renal
pelvis

Kidney

Cancer in the
renal pelvis

Parts removed

Ureter

Bladder

Prostate

Urethra

Percutaneous nephrolithotomy

- If you regularly lose too much water from your body or do not drink enough fluids, you will become dehydrated. Your urine will be too concentrated and cause calcium crystals in the urine to form stones (calculi) in the kidney. Some people are born with a tendency to form stones.

- Percutaneous nephrolithotomy is an operation to remove kidney stones.

- The operation involves making a 'track' down to the kidney through a 1–2 cm skin incision. This track is widened until it is similar in size to a large ball-point pen. A special telescope called a nephroscope is inserted along the track so that the surgeon can see the stone. The stone is then either removed whole or, if large, broken into pieces that are taken out separately using special instruments.

- The operation is performed under a general anaesthetic and usually takes about 1 hour.

- During the operation, a catheter is passed up the urethra into the bladder and another tube is inserted to drain the wound. The catheter and drainage tube will be removed after 24–48 hours. After the operation, you may feel a little sore in your side and pass some blood in your urine.

- The average hospital stay is 2–3 days and you can usually return to work within 10 days.

- Increasing your non-alcoholic fluid intake to more than 2 litres/day may help stop stones reforming.

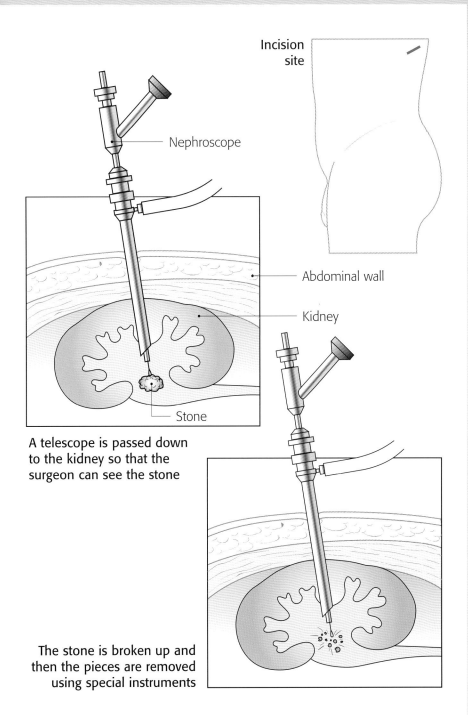

Incision
site

Nephroscope

Abdominal wall

Kidney

Stone

A telescope is passed down
to the kidney so that the
surgeon can see the stone

The stone is broken up and
then the pieces are removed
using special instruments

Open nephrolithotomy

- If you regularly lose too much water from your body or do not drink enough fluids, you will become dehydrated. Your urine will be too concentrated and cause calcium crystals in the urine to form stones (calculi) in the kidney. Some people are born with a tendency to form stones.

- Open nephrolithotomy is an operation to remove very large stones (called 'staghorn' calculi because of their shape) and stones that cannot be broken up.

- The operation involves either simply lifting out the stone using forceps or breaking it up and then removing the pieces. You will need an X-ray to check that all of the stone has been removed.

- The procedure is carried out under a general anaesthetic and may take several hours.

- During the operation, a catheter is passed up the urethra into the bladder and a drainage tube is inserted into the wound. The catheter and drainage tube will usually be removed after 2–4 days. After the operation, you may feel some discomfort in your side but this can be controlled with painkillers.

- The average hospital stay is 7–10 days, but complete recovery takes several months. You will need to visit the clinic again after about 3 months for more X-rays and scans to check that stones have not reformed.

- Increasing your non-alcoholic fluid intake to more than 2 litres/day may help stop stones reforming.

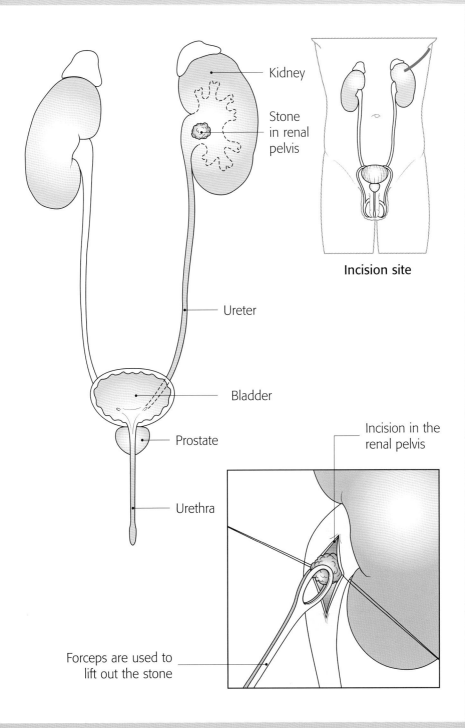

Kidney

Stone
in renal
pelvis

Incision site

Ureter

Bladder

Prostate

Incision in the
renal pelvis

Urethra

Forceps are used to
lift out the stone

Lithotripsy of kidney stone

- If you regularly lose too much water from your body or do not drink enough fluids, you will become dehydrated. Your urine will be too concentrated and cause calcium crystals in the urine to form stones (calculi) in the kidney. Some people are born with a tendency to form stones.

- Extracorporeal shock wave lithotripsy (ESWL) is a technique used to break up stones without surgery.

- ESWL uses shock waves that are generated outside the body and then focused onto the stone to break it up. The pieces are flushed out of the kidney in the urine.

- No anaesthetic is needed for the procedure. You will be asked to lie on a special couch and the exact position of the stone will be found, using ultrasound or X-rays, so that the shock waves can be focused onto it.

- Up to 5000 individual shocks are then given over about 1 hour. The shocks feel uncomfortable rather than painful and you may feel a little sore for a few days.

- After the procedure, you will be asked to drink plenty of fluids to help flush away any remaining pieces of stone.

- You will need to visit the clinic again for more X-rays to check that all the pieces of stone have been passed in your urine and that no new stones have formed.

- Increasing your non-alcoholic fluid intake to more than 2 litres/day may help stop stones reforming.

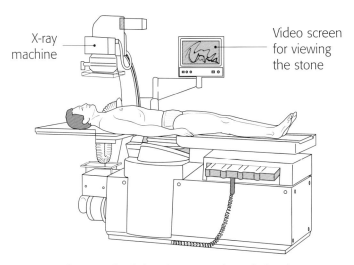

X-ray machine

Video screen for viewing the stone

The patient lies on the lithotripter couch and shock waves are delivered from the back. X-rays or ultrasound are used to focus the shock waves onto the stone

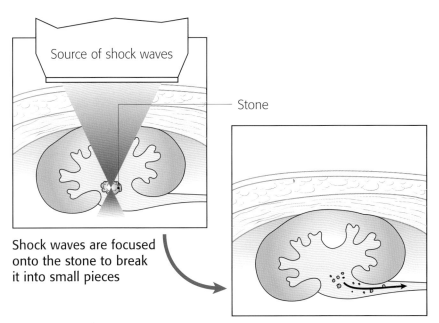

Source of shock waves

Stone

Shock waves are focused onto the stone to break it into small pieces

The pieces are flushed out of the body in the urine

Open removal of ureteric stone

- If you regularly lose too much water from your body or do not drink enough fluids, you will become dehydrated. Your urine will be too concentrated and cause calcium crystals in the urine to form stones (calculi) in the kidney. Some people are born with a tendency to form stones.

- Occasionally, a stone lodges in the ureter and cannot be removed telescopically or broken up by shock-wave treatment. If this happens, open removal through a skin incision may be necessary.

- The operation is performed under a general anaesthetic and usually takes $1-1^1/_2$ hours.

- During the operation, the stone is lifted out through an incision in the ureter. Also, a catheter is passed up the urethra into the bladder and a drainage tube is inserted into the wound. The catheter and drainage tube will usually be removed after 2–3 days.

- After the operation, you may feel some discomfort in your side but this can be controlled with painkillers. The average hospital stay is 5–7 days, but complete recovery may take 4–6 weeks.

- Increasing your non-alcoholic fluid intake to more than 2 litres/day may help stop stones reforming.

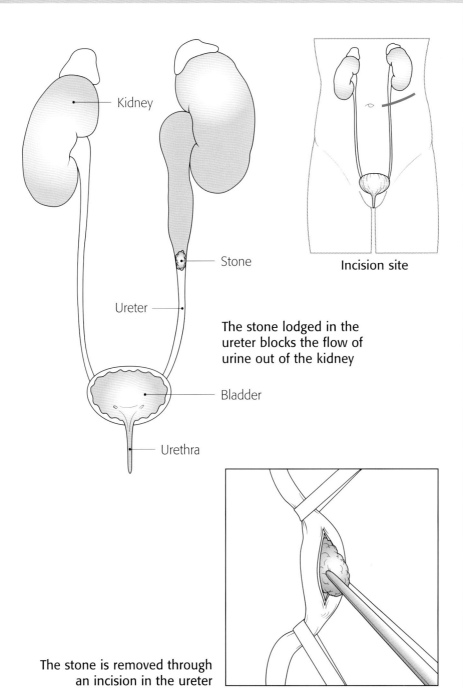

Kidney

Stone

Ureter

The stone lodged in the ureter blocks the flow of urine out of the kidney

Bladder

Urethra

Incision site

The stone is removed through an incision in the ureter

Ureteroscopic stone removal

- If you regularly lose too much water from your body or do not drink enough fluids, you will become dehydrated. Your urine will be too concentrated and cause calcium crystals in the urine to form stones (calculi) in the kidney. Some people are born with a tendency to form stones.

- Stones that pass down the ureter often lodge at the lower end where the ureter is narrowest as it enters the bladder. These stones are usually removed using a specialized narrow 'telescope' called a ureteroscope.

- The ureteroscope is passed up the urethra into the bladder and from there into the ureter. Next, the stone is trapped in a wire 'basket', and the telescope, basket and stone all removed together. Larger stones may be broken up before removal. A tube called a 'stent' may be left in the ureter for a few weeks to allow pieces of stone to pass out in the urine or the ureter to heal.

- The procedure is performed under a general anaesthetic and takes 20–40 minutes. X-rays may be taken to help the surgeon perform the operation.

- After stone removal, a catheter is passed up the urethra into the bladder. This will be removed after about 12 hours. You may feel some discomfort after the operation but this can be controlled with painkillers.

- You will usually need to stay in hospital overnight, but can resume normal activities within a few days. Increasing your non-alcoholic fluid intake to more than 2 litres/day may help stop stones reforming.

The ureteroscope is passed up the urethra
through the bladder and into the ureter

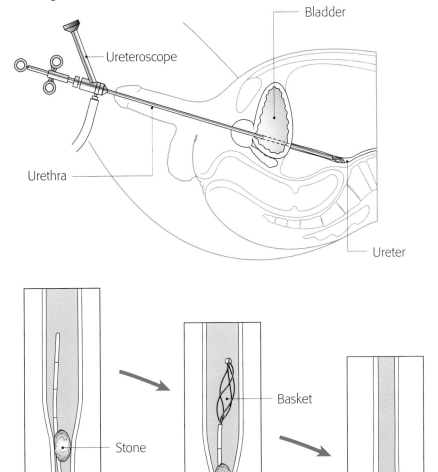

The stone is trapped in a 'basket' and then the
ureteroscope, basket and stone are removed together

Lithotripsy of lower ureteric stone

- If you regularly lose too much water from your body or do not drink enough fluids, you will become dehydrated. Your urine will be too concentrated and cause calcium crystals in the urine to form stones (calculi) in the kidney. Some people are born with a tendency to form stones.

- Stones that pass down the ureter often lodge at the lower end where the ureter is narrowest as it enters the bladder. If this happens, urine cannot flow freely from the kidney and this may cause severe pain (renal colic).

- Though extracorporeal shock wave lithotripsy (ESWL) is most suitable for breaking up stones in the kidney, it can also be used to break up stones that are lodged elsewhere. ESWL involves using shock waves to break up the stone into small pieces which are then flushed out of the kidney in the urine.

- No anaesthetic is needed for the procedure. You will be asked to lie on a special couch and the exact position of the stone will be found, using ultrasound or X-rays, so that the shock waves can be focused onto it.

- Usually, between 2000 and 5000 shocks are given over about 1 hour. The shocks feel uncomfortable rather than painful and you may feel a little sore for a few days.

- After the procedure, you will be asked to drink plenty of fluids to help flush out any remaining pieces of stone.

- Increasing your non-alcoholic fluid intake to more than 2 litres/day may help stop stones reforming.

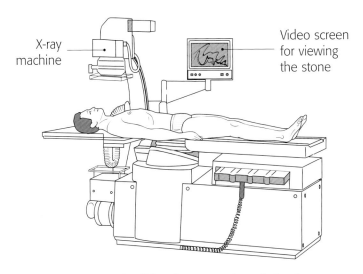

X-ray machine

Video screen for viewing the stone

The patient lies on the lithotripter couch and shock waves are delivered from the back. X-rays or ultrasound are used to focus the shock waves onto the stone

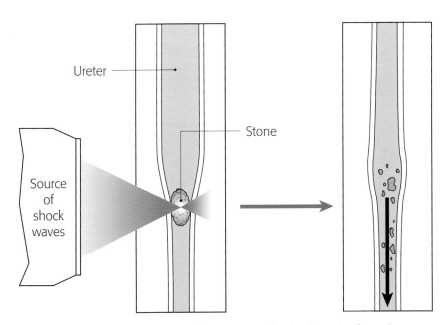

Ureter

Stone

Source of shock waves

The stone is broken up and pieces are flushed out in the urine

Flexible cystoscopy

- Cystoscopy is examination of the lining of the bladder using a 'telescope' about the thickness of a pen called a cystoscope. There are two types of cystoscope – flexible and rigid.

- Flexible cystoscopy is usually performed to find out the cause of a symptom, such as blood in the urine (haematuria).

- Local anaesthetic gel is inserted into the urethra. The flexible cystoscope is then passed up the urethra and into the bladder. The inside of the bladder is carefully examined to identify stones, bladder tumours or other abnormalities. Tiny tissue samples (biopsies) may also be taken. If more investigations or surgery are needed, you may need to have a rigid cystoscopy later.

- Flexible cystoscopy takes only a few minutes and is usually performed as a day-case procedure.

- After the examination, you may feel a little discomfort when passing urine, but this should settle within a day or so. You will be asked to drink extra fluids for 24 hours and may be given antibiotics to help reduce the risk of urinary infection.

- If you develop a temperature or symptoms of cystitis, you should consult your doctor because you may need to take a full course of antibiotics.

Men

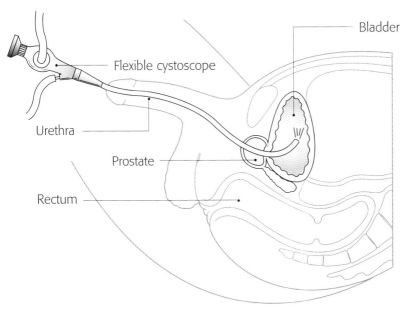

Bladder

Flexible cystoscope

Urethra

Prostate

Rectum

Women

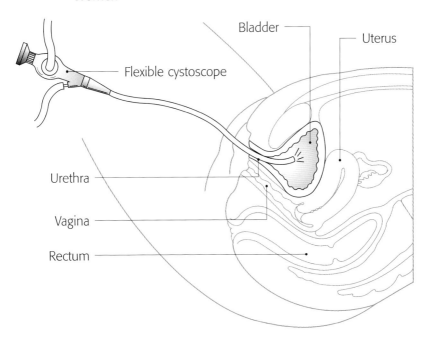

Bladder

Uterus

Flexible cystoscope

Urethra

Vagina

Rectum

Rigid cystoscopy

- Cystoscopy is examination of the lining of the bladder using a thin 'telescope' called a cystoscope. There are two types of cystoscope – rigid and flexible.

- Rigid cystoscopy can be performed under a local anaesthetic. However, men usually prefer to be sedated or have a light general anaesthetic because the male urethra is longer and more curved than in females and this makes the procedure a little more uncomfortable. The examination takes only a few minutes.

- The rigid cystoscope is passed up the urethra and into the bladder. The inside of the bladder is carefully examined to identify stones, tumours or other abnormalities. Various minor procedures can be performed at the same time, for example taking tissue samples (biopsies) or destroying abnormal tissue with heat (diathermy).

- The examination is usually performed as a day-case procedure, but you may need to stay in hospital overnight if other bladder investigations are carried out.

- After the procedure, you may feel a little discomfort when passing urine, but this should settle within a day or so. You will be asked to drink extra fluids for 24 hours and may be given antibiotics to help reduce the risk of infection.

- If you develop a temperature or symptoms of cystitis, you should consult your doctor because you may need to take a full course of antibiotics.

Men

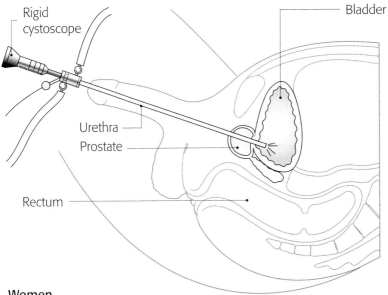

Rigid cystoscope

Bladder

Urethra

Prostate

Rectum

Women

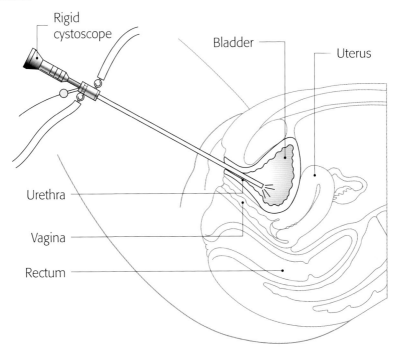

Rigid cystoscope

Bladder

Uterus

Urethra

Vagina

Rectum

Bladder stone removal (lithopaxy)

- If you regularly lose too much water from your body or do not drink enough fluids, you will become dehydrated. Your urine will be too concentrated and cause calcium crystals in the urine to form stones (calculi) in the bladder. Some people are born with a tendency to form stones.

- Bladder stones are usually removed using a 'telescope' called a cystoscope. Stones can be removed whole or broken into pieces which are then taken out separately.

- The procedure is usually performed under a light general anaesthetic and takes 20–30 minutes.

- During the operation, a catheter is passed up the urethra into the bladder. The catheter will be removed after about 12–24 hours. After the procedure, you may feel a little discomfort when passing urine, but this should settle within a day or so.

- You may need to visit the clinic again once or twice for X-rays to check that all the pieces of stone have been removed and that no new stones have formed.

- If a stone is very large, or associated with another abnormality such as an enlarged prostate, open removal of the stone through a cut in the lower abdomen may be necessary.

- Increasing your non-alcoholic fluid intake to more than 2 litres/day may help stop stones reforming. If stone formation is associated with prostate enlargement, you may need treatment with drugs or surgery.

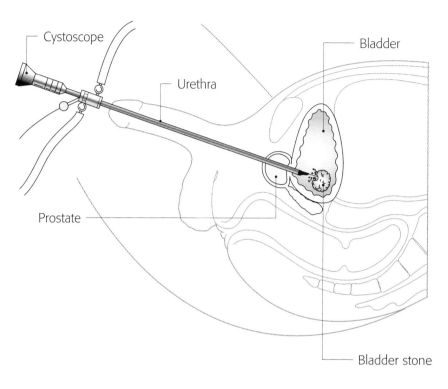

Cystoscope

Bladder

Urethra

Prostate

Bladder stone

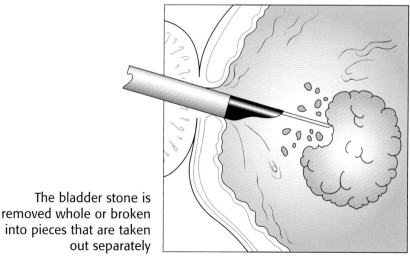

The bladder stone is removed whole or broken into pieces that are taken out separately

Transurethral resection of bladder tumour (TURBT)

- Transurethral resection of bladder tumour (TURBT) is a treatment for bladder cancer.

- The operation involves passing an instrument called a resectoscope up the urethra and into the bladder.

- The bladder tumour is then cut away and removed in pieces. The tissue is examined microscopically to find out how far the cancer cells have invaded the muscle of the bladder wall.

- The operation is performed under a light general anaesthetic and usually takes 10–20 minutes.

- At the end of the operation, a catheter is passed up the urethra into the bladder. The catheter will be removed after 12–24 hours. Some bleeding into the urine may occur during this time, which will be flushed out with fluid put into the bladder through the catheter. The average hospital stay is 2–3 days, but will depend on how much surgery was necessary.

- The need for further treatment will depend on what is seen when the pieces of tumour are examined under the microscope. If the tumour has not spread, regular cystoscopy is usually all that is needed to check that the cancer is not growing again. In other cases, a course of medicine instilled into the bladder, radiotherapy or sometimes surgery may be needed.

- If the cancer recurs frequently, anticancer drugs may be put into the bladder after the operation to kill any remaining cancer cells and help stop further recurrence.

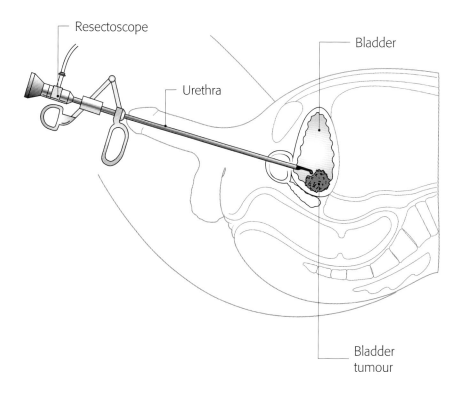

Resectoscope

Urethra

Bladder

Bladder
tumour

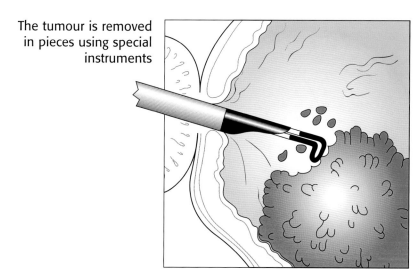

The tumour is removed
in pieces using special
instruments

Radical cystectomy with ileal loop diversion

- Radical cystectomy with ileal loop diversion is an operation to treat bladder cancer that either recurs after radiotherapy or for which radiotherapy is unlikely to be effective.

- The operation involves removing the entire bladder, usually the local lymph glands, and sometimes the urethra. In men, the prostate gland is removed as well.

- The operation is carried out under a general anaesthetic and usually takes 3–4 hours.

- To allow urine to leave your body, a permanent artificial opening on the abdomen called a stoma is made using a small part of the intestine, which is then joined to the ureters. In future, your urine will drain into a changeable bag attached to the skin of your abdomen. The bag will need to be emptied regularly.

- During the operation, a tube will be inserted to drain the wound and a bag attached to drain the urine.

- After the operation, any discomfort can be controlled with painkillers. You will not be able to eat or drink for several days until the join in the intestine has healed. When you are well enough, a 'stomatherapist' will teach you how to care for your stoma and manage the bags.

- The average hospital stay is usually 10–14 days and complete recovery may take 4–6 months. You will need to visit the clinic after 3 months to check that the operation has been a success, and then at 6-monthly intervals.

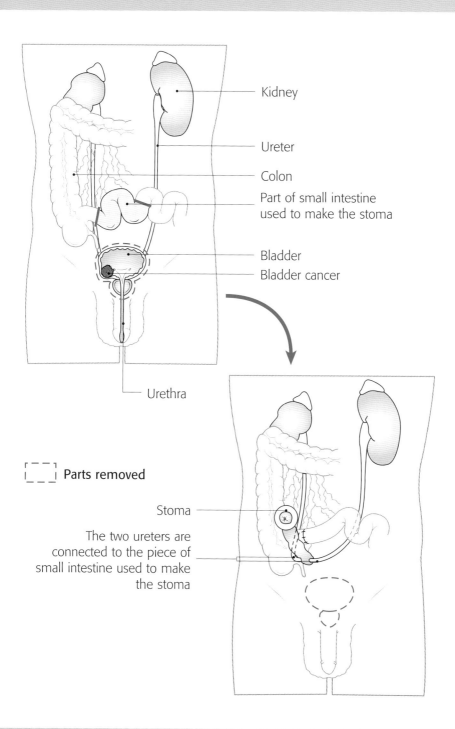

Kidney

Ureter

Colon

Part of small intestine
used to make the stoma

Bladder
Bladder cancer

Urethra

Parts removed

Stoma

The two ureters are
connected to the piece of
small intestine used to make
the stoma

Radical cystectomy with total bladder replacement

- Radical cystectomy with total bladder replacement is an operation to treat bladder cancer that is invading the bladder wall. It may be suitable for younger, fitter patients and, because bladder cancer is more common in men and the male urethra is less likely to leak, it is more commonly performed in men than in women.

- The operation involves removing the bladder, the local lymph glands and, in men, the prostate gland. A new bladder is constructed using a piece of small intestine, and then the two ureters and urethra are joined to it. The operation is performed under a general anaesthetic and takes 4–6 hours.

- During the operation, drainage tubes are placed into the bladder and kidneys to allow the new bladder to heal before it fills with urine. After the operation, any discomfort can be controlled with painkillers.

- The average hospital stay is usually 12–16 days, but complete recovery often takes 3–6 months.

- After surgery, some patients leak urine, especially at night, and you may need to learn to pass a catheter up the urethra regularly to empty the new bladder fully. It is also normal to pass some mucus in your urine. The mucus is secreted by the piece of small intestine that was used to form the new bladder and is usually harmless.

- You will need to visit the clinic after 3 months to check that the operation has been a success, and then again at 6-monthly intervals to have blood tests and an X-ray.

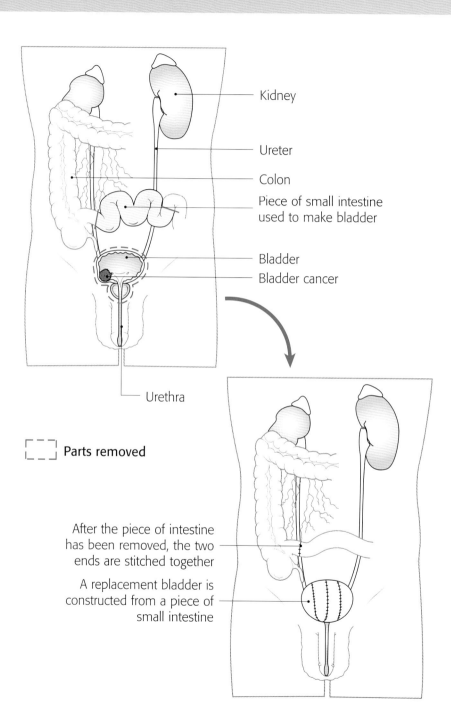

Kidney

Ureter

Colon

Piece of small intestine
used to make bladder

Bladder

Bladder cancer

Urethra

┌──┐
└──┘ **Parts removed**

After the piece of intestine
has been removed, the two
ends are stitched together

A replacement bladder is
constructed from a piece of
small intestine

'Clam' ileocystoplasty

- 'Clam' ileocystoplasty is an operation used to enlarge a shrunken or overactive (and sometimes both) bladder that has not responded to less invasive treatments, such as bladder training or drug therapy.

- The bladder is opened, like a clam, to reveal the inside. A piece of small intestine is then used to enlarge the bladder.

- The operation is performed under a general anaesthetic and takes 1–2 hours.

- During the operation, a catheter is passed up the urethra into the bladder and left in place for 7–10 days to keep the bladder empty while it heals. You may feel some discomfort after the operation, but this can be controlled with painkillers.

- The average hospital stay is about 10 days, but complete recovery may take 3–4 months.

- The enlarged bladder cannot contract as well as a healthy one to push the urine into the urethra and out of the body. For this reason, you may need to learn to pass a thin catheter up the urethra regularly to empty your bladder fully.

- It is also normal to pass some mucus in your urine. The mucus is secreted by the piece of small intestine that was used to enlarge the bladder and is usually harmless. Drinking extra fluids will help you to pass the mucus more easily.

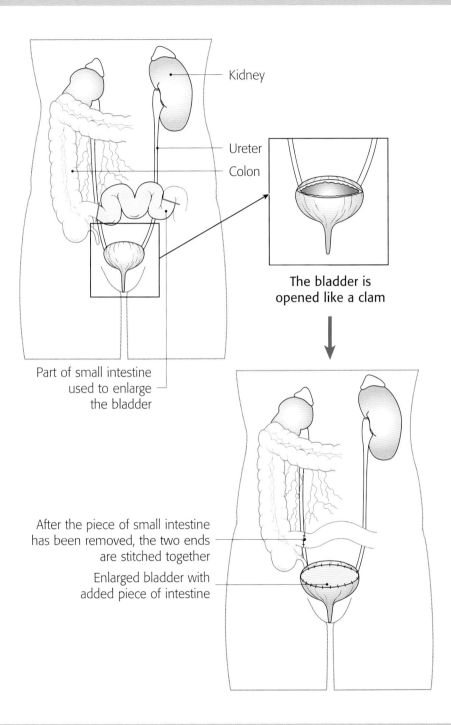

Kidney

Ureter
Colon

The bladder is
opened like a clam

Part of small intestine
used to enlarge
the bladder

After the piece of small intestine
has been removed, the two ends
are stitched together

Enlarged bladder with
added piece of intestine

Transurethral resection of the prostate (TURP)

- Transurethral resection of the prostate (TURP for short) is an operation to treat urinary problems caused by an enlarged and obstructing prostate. An instrument called a 'resectoscope' is passed through the penis and up the urethra. The middle of the enlarged prostate is then cut away and the pieces removed from the bladder and sent to the laboratory.

- The operation is performed under a general anaesthetic and usually takes 30–60 minutes.

- At the end of the operation, a catheter is passed up the urethra into the bladder to drain off the urine. The catheter can also be used to flush out the bladder with fluid and will be removed after 36–48 hours. After the operation, you should feel only mild discomfort but you may notice some blood in your urine on and off for several days or even weeks.

- The average hospital stay is 3–4 days, but you will need to 'take it easy' for a few weeks.

- After surgery, the flow with which urine is passed usually improves rapidly. However, you may need to urinate frequently and feel a burning sensation on passing urine, but this should improve after a few weeks.

- Most men develop permanent 'retrograde ejaculation' after TURP. Semen passes into the bladder during orgasm instead of out of the penis. This is not harmful and the semen will come out the next time you pass urine. Erections, sex drive and the sensation of orgasm are not usually affected.

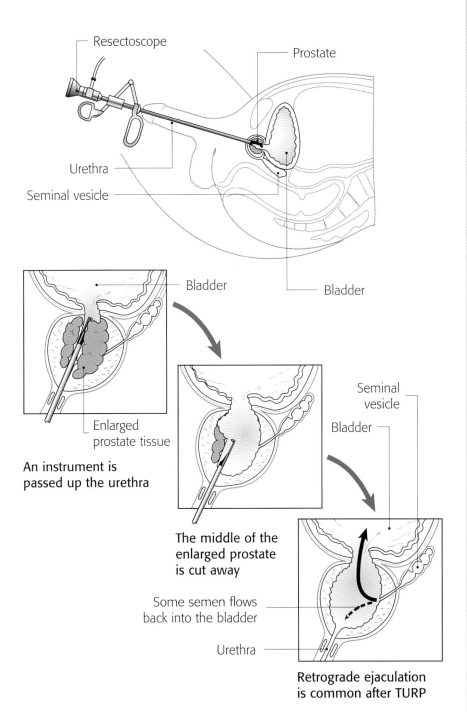

Resectoscope

Prostate

Urethra

Seminal vesicle

Bladder

Bladder

Enlarged
prostate tissue

**An instrument is
passed up the urethra**

**The middle of the
enlarged prostate
is cut away**

Seminal
vesicle

Bladder

Some semen flows
back into the bladder

Urethra

**Retrograde ejaculation
is common after TURP**

© Health Press Limited

Transurethral incision of the prostate (TUIP)

- Transurethral incision of the prostate (TUIP for short) is an operation to treat urinary problems caused by a small, but obstructing prostate or a tight bladder neck.

- In TUIP, an instrument the thickness of a pen called a 'resectoscope' is passed through the penis and up the urethra. One or two small cuts are then made in the bladder neck and prostate. These cuts allow the prostate tissue and bladder neck around the urethra to spring apart. This reduces the pressure of the prostate on the urethra and makes it easier to pass urine.

- The operation is performed under a general anaesthetic and usually takes 15–25 minutes.

- During the operation, a catheter will be passed up the urethra into the bladder to drain off urine. The catheter can also be used to flush out the bladder with fluid and will be removed after 24 hours.

- The average hospital stay is 2–3 days, but you will need to 'take it easy' for 1–2 weeks to reduce the risk of bleeding.

- After the operation, most people find that symptoms and urine flow improve. Up to 15% of patients develop permanent 'retrograde ejaculation'. Semen passes into the bladder during orgasm instead of out of the penis. This is not harmful and the semen will come out the next time you pass urine. Erections, sex drive and the sensation of orgasm are not usually affected.

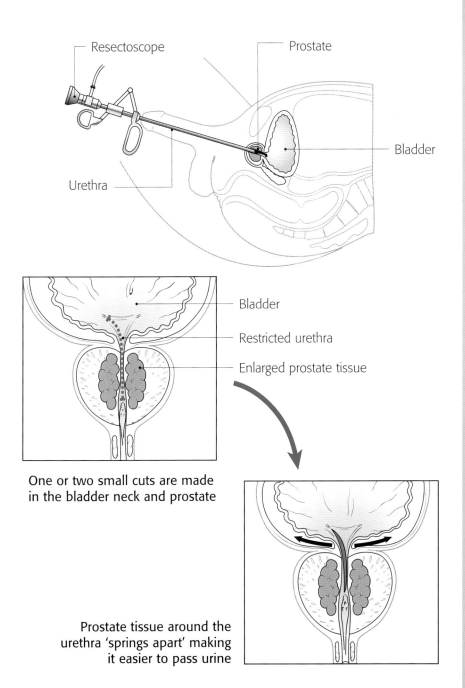

Resectoscope

Prostate

Bladder

Urethra

Bladder

Restricted urethra

Enlarged prostate tissue

One or two small cuts are made
in the bladder neck and prostate

Prostate tissue around the
urethra 'springs apart' making
it easier to pass urine

Laser therapy to the prostate

- Laser therapy can be used to treat urinary problems caused by an enlarged prostate. Laser energy is used to destroy some of the prostate tissue by intense local heat.

- The procedure is carried out under a general anaesthetic and takes about 20 minutes. A laser probe is inserted up the urethra and the prostate tissue is then treated with the laser.

- Bleeding after laser therapy is rare, but the treated area usually feels sore and you will probably feel a burning sensation when passing urine for about 4 weeks. Urinary tract infections (UTIs) may also occur.

- After the operation, a catheter will be passed up the urethra into the bladder to drain off the urine. This will usually be removed after a few days, but you may need a catheter for longer.

- The average hospital stay is 1–2 days. If you continue to use a catheter at home, you will probably need to return to hospital to have it removed and for an ultrasound examination to check that your bladder is emptying properly.

- About 30% of patients develop permanent 'retrograde ejaculation' after laser therapy. Semen passes into the bladder during orgasm instead of out of the penis. This is not harmful and the semen will come out the next time you pass urine. Impotence (inability to have an erection) is very uncommon, and both problems occur less often than after conventional prostate surgery.

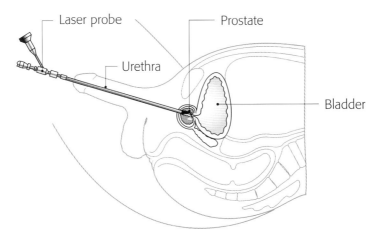

Laser probe — Prostate

Urethra

Bladder

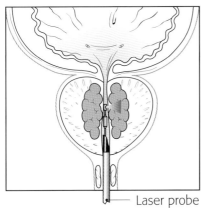

Laser energy destroys prostate tissue without bleeding

Laser probe

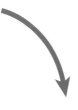

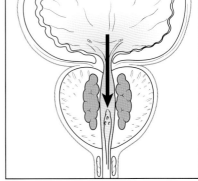

The prostate no longer presses on the urethra making it easier to pass urine

Retropubic prostatectomy (RPP)

- Retropubic prostatectomy (RPP for short) is an operation that is usually performed only if the prostate is too large to be removed telescopically.

- In RPP, the central part of the prostate is removed through a cut in the lower abdomen. The cut will therefore leave a scar.

- The procedure is carried out under a general anaesthetic and usually takes less than 1 hour.

- During the operation, a catheter will be passed up the urethra into the bladder to drain off the urine. This will be removed after 3–4 days.

- You will be able to go home about 1 week after surgery, but will need to rest for 4–6 weeks and avoid heavy lifting. You may also notice some blood in your urine for 10–14 days or more after the operation.

- Most patients experience an immediate improvement in the flow of urine. However, you may need to urinate frequently, and sometimes urgently, and will feel a burning sensation on passing urine for a few weeks or even months.

- The pieces of the prostate removed during surgery will be examined under the microscope to check that no prostate cancer is present.

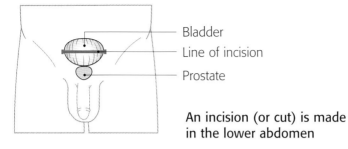

22

Bladder

Line of incision

Prostate

An incision (or cut) is made
in the lower abdomen

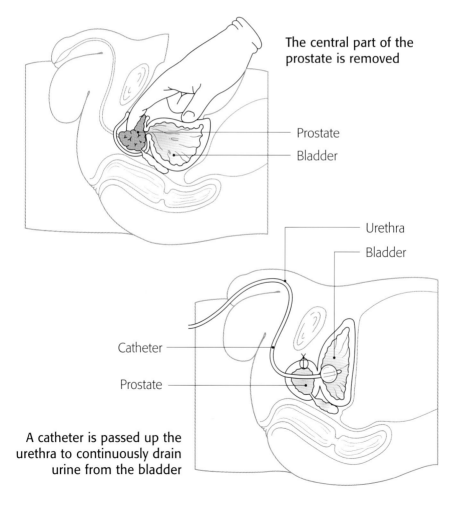

The central part of the
prostate is removed

Prostate

Bladder

Urethra

Bladder

Catheter

Prostate

A catheter is passed up the
urethra to continuously drain
urine from the bladder

Radical prostatectomy

- Radical prostatectomy is an operation to remove prostate cancer if it has not spread to other parts of the body. The prostate, with the tumour, and the seminal vesicles are removed through a cut in the lower abdomen and sent to the laboratory for analysis. The operation is done under a general anaesthetic and takes 1–3 hours.

- During the operation, a catheter will be passed up the urethra into the bladder to drain off urine. You will usually need to return to hospital to have the catheter removed after 2–3 weeks.

- After the operation, any discomfort can be controlled with painkillers and you can normally go home after 5–7 days. Complete recovery takes 6–8 weeks, but you may feel tired for several months and should avoid heavy lifting.

- At first, you may leak urine when coughing or moving but there is only a small (less than 3%) risk of persistent incontinence after surgery. However, there is more than a 50% chance of impotence (inability to have an erection) but this can often be treated with tablets or injections.

- If all of the prostate cancer is removed successfully, the level of prostate-specific antigen (PSA for short) in your blood will fall to zero and remain undetectable.

- You will need to visit the clinic every 3–6 months for blood tests. If the PSA level rises, this usually means that cancer is still present or has recurred. A quarter to one-third of patients will require further treatment with radiotherapy or hormone therapy.

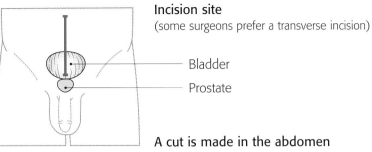

23

Incision site
(some surgeons prefer a transverse incision)

Bladder

Prostate

A cut is made in the abdomen

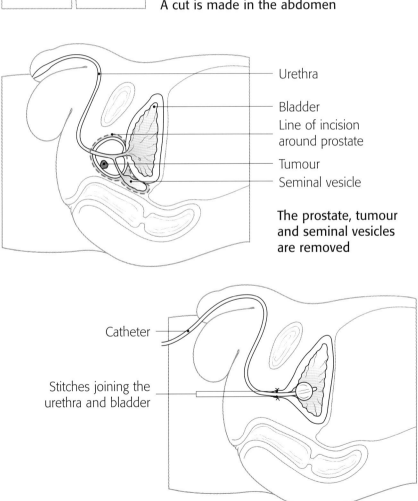

Urethra

Bladder
Line of incision
around prostate

Tumour
Seminal vesicle

**The prostate, tumour
and seminal vesicles
are removed**

Catheter

Stitches joining the
urethra and bladder

**The urethra is joined to the
bladder and a catheter is inserted**

Urethrotomy

- In men, the urethra is likely to suffer scarring after a urethral infection or procedures that involve passing instruments up the urethra. Scar tissue can narrow the urethra and obstruct the flow of urine. If this happens, you will have a weak stream and need to urinate frequently.

- Urethrotomy involves passing an instrument called a urethrotome through the penis and up the urethra. A small cut is then made in the narrowed part of the urethra to widen it.

- The operation is performed under a general anaesthetic and takes 10–20 minutes.

- During the operation, a catheter will be passed up the urethra into the bladder to drain off the urine. The catheter will usually be removed after 12–24 hours. After the operation, there should be only mild discomfort but you may feel a burning sensation when you pass urine for a few days.

- You will need to learn how to pass a catheter up the urethra regularly to stop it narrowing again.

- Short-term results are usually good, but the narrowing may eventually recur. If this happens, you will need to have either another urethrotomy or an operation called a urethroplasty to permanently repair the defect.

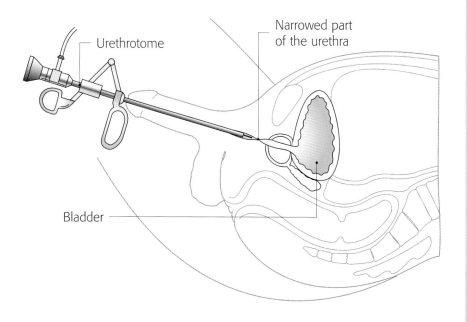

24

Urethrotome

Narrowed part
of the urethra

Bladder

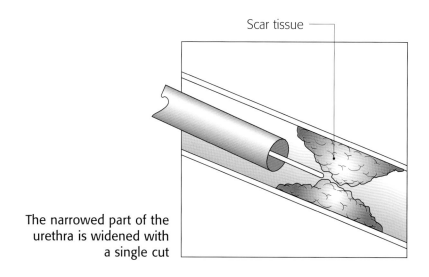

Scar tissue

The narrowed part of the
urethra is widened with
a single cut

Urethroplasty

- In men, the urethra is likely to suffer scarring after a urethral infection or procedures that involve passing instruments up the urethra. Scar tissue can narrow the urethra and obstruct the flow of urine. If this happens, you will have a weak stream and need to urinate frequently.

- If a narrowing or 'stricture' of the urethra recurs, you may need an operation called a urethroplasty to repair the damaged area.

- The damaged section of the urethra is removed through a skin incision beneath the scrotum (the perineum). The two healthy ends of the urethra are then joined over a temporary tube called a catheter. Sometimes, an additional skin graft is required.

- The operation is performed under a general anaesthetic and takes 1–2 hours.

- The catheter inserted during the operation will usually be left in place for 2 weeks. Before the catheter is removed, an X-ray will be taken to check that the urethra has healed properly.

- After the operation, you should feel only a little discomfort, but may find having a catheter for 2 weeks inconvenient.

- Urethroplasty is usually extremely successful and further surgery is rarely necessary.

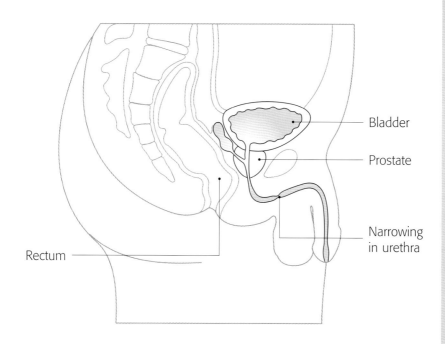

25

Bladder

Prostate

Narrowing in urethra

Rectum

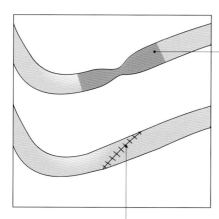

The narrowed section of the urethra is removed

Catheter

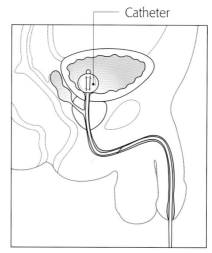

Stitches join the two healthy ends of the urethra together

During the operation, a catheter is inserted to allow the urethra to heal

Colposuspension or sling procedure

- Colposuspension is an open operation to treat 'stress incontinence', which is leakage of urine on coughing or sneezing. It is caused by a weakness in the bladder neck and pelvic floor and is common in women who have had several babies delivered vaginally.

- In women, the operation involves raising the bladder and urethra by inserting several stitches through the vagina on each side, and then attaching them to the pelvic bone.

- The operation is performed through a cut in the abdomen under a general anaesthetic and takes 1–2 hours.

- During the operation, a catheter is inserted through a small incision in the abdomen into the bladder to drain off the urine.

- The catheter will be 'clamped off' daily to allow the bladder to fill so that you can attempt to pass urine normally. If this is not possible, the clamp is released to drain the urine and the process is repeated the following day. When urine can be passed normally, usually after 4–5 days, the catheter will be removed.

- The average hospital stay is 7–10 days and you can usually resume normal activities after 6–8 weeks. The overall success rate of the operation is more than 80%.

- The 'sling procedure' is a new alternative operation to colposuspension. Three small incisions are made and a sling is used to raise the bladder and urethra to prevent urine leaking out.

26

Colposuspension

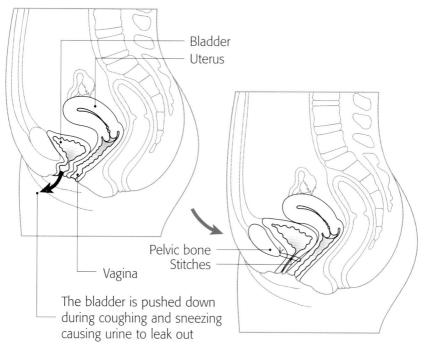

Bladder
Uterus

Pelvic bone
Stitches

Vagina

The bladder is pushed down
during coughing and sneezing
causing urine to leak out

Sling procedure

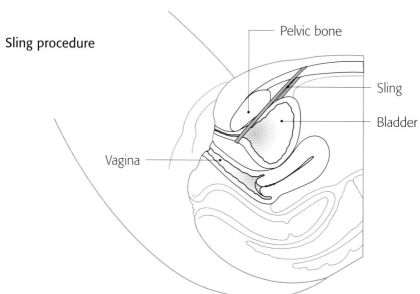

Pelvic bone

Sling

Bladder

Vagina

Circumcision

- Circumcision is often performed for social or religious reasons in children or babies. In older individuals, the operation is done only for medical reasons, such as scarring or inability to pull back the foreskin.

- The operation involves the removal of the foreskin of the penis which leaves the head or 'glans' of the penis exposed.

- The operation is performed under a general anaesthetic and takes 20–30 minutes.

- After the operation, you will have some soreness but this lasts for only a few days and can be easily controlled with painkillers. In mature men, sexual intercourse should be avoided for 3–4 weeks until the skin is completely healed.

- The operation is usually performed as a day-case procedure and you or your child will usually be able to go home the same day.

- Self-dissolving stitches, which do not need to be removed, are used to bring the skin edges together.

- You will usually need to visit the clinic again 6–12 weeks after the operation to check that healing is satisfactory.

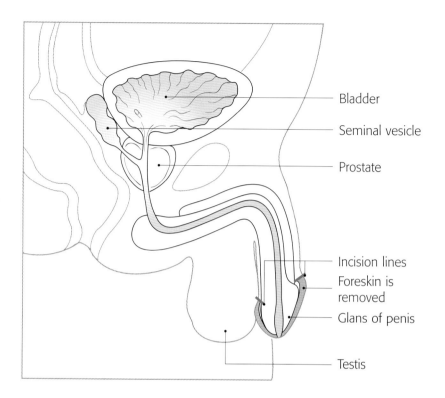

27

- Bladder
- Seminal vesicle
- Prostate
- Incision lines
- Foreskin is removed
- Glans of penis
- Testis

Before surgery

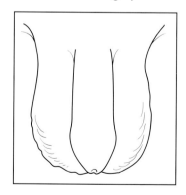

After surgery

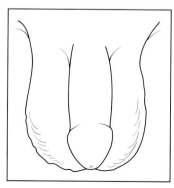

Vasectomy

- A vasectomy is an operation used to sterilize men. It should be undertaken only after careful thought and discussion with your partner. It should be generally considered irreversible, though sometimes a successful reversal operation is possible.

- Sterilization is achieved by cutting the two tubes that carry the semen from the testes (testicles) to the urethra. These tubes are called the vas deferens.

- The operation involves making two small incisions in the scrotum. A segment of the vas deferens is then removed on either side and sent to the pathology laboratory to confirm that the correct structure has been divided. Each incision is then closed with self-dissolving stitches.

- The operation is performed under a local or light general anaesthetic and takes 10–15 minutes.

- After the operation, you will feel only mild discomfort but it is a good idea to 'take it easy' for 24–48 hours.

- The operation is more than 99% effective, but can occasionally fail if the two ends of the vas rejoin spontaneously. If this happens, it usually does so within 3 months, but very occasionally the ends may rejoin later.

- About 3 months after the operation, a sperm count is usually done to check that sterility has been achieved. If sperm are still present, the test is repeated in a few months time. An alternative method of contraception should be used until sterilization is confirmed by a negative count.

28

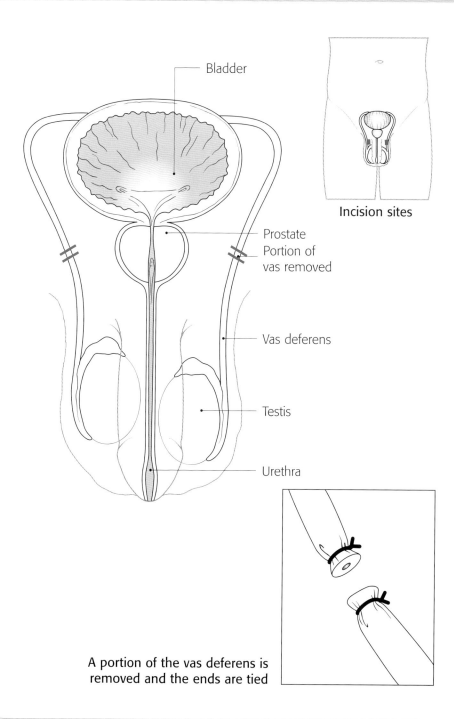

Bladder

Prostate
Portion of
vas removed

Vas deferens

Testis

Urethra

Incision sites

A portion of the vas deferens is
removed and the ends are tied

Reversal of vasectomy

- A vasectomy is an operation used to sterilize men. It is sometimes reversible. The chance of having a successful vasectomy reversal decreases as you get older and the time since the original operation increases.

- The operation involves making an incision in the scrotum. The two ends of the vas deferens (the tube that carries semen from the testicles to the urethra) are then located and carefully rejoined. This is done on both sides.

- The operation is performed under a general anaesthetic, takes at least 1 hour, and can be done safely as a day-case procedure.

- After the operation, you may feel mild discomfort and should 'take it easy' for a few days.

- Overall, the operation can restore sperm to semen in more than 50% of patients. However, not all of these patients will be able to make their partner pregnant. The longer the time since the original vasectomy operation, the greater the chance that sperm quality will be permanently impaired.

- A sperm count is usually performed at 3 months to find out whether the operation has been successful.

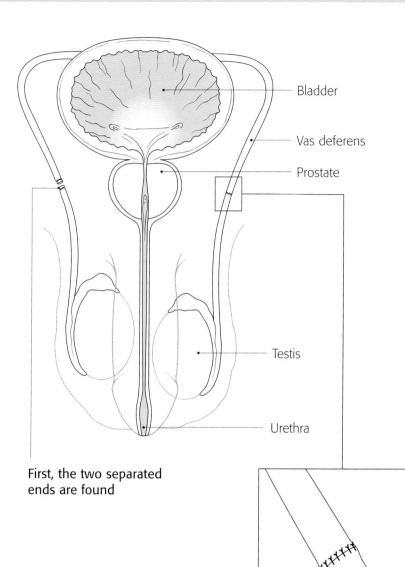

29

Bladder

Vas deferens

Prostate

Testis

Urethra

First, the two separated
ends are found

Second, the ends are prepared and
carefully stitched together

Excision of hydrocele

- A hydrocele is a collection of fluid that develops around the testis (testicle) and produces a lump in the scrotum. The swelling usually develops very gradually.

- The condition is harmless and surgery is needed only if the swelling is uncomfortable or is increasing in size.

- The operation involves making an incision in the scrotum, removing the fluid and then either stitching the lining of the hydrocele around the back of the testis or cutting it out. The wound is then closed with self-dissolving stitches.

- The operation is usually performed under a light, general anaesthetic and takes 20–30 minutes.

- After surgery, you may feel mild discomfort but this can be controlled with painkillers. Your scrotum and the affected testis may be swollen for several months.

- The operation is usually performed as a day-case procedure, so you can normally go home the same day. However, you should 'take it easy' for a few days because there is a small risk of bruising and swelling.

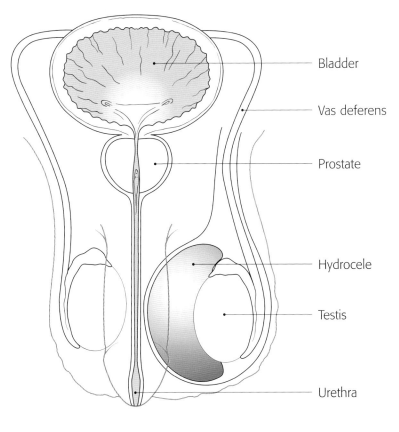

30

Bladder

Vas deferens

Prostate

Hydrocele

Testis

Urethra

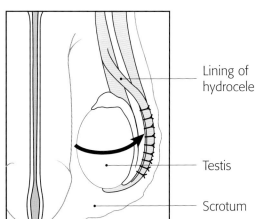

Lining of
hydrocele

Testis

Scrotum

The fluid is removed
and the lining of the
hydrocele is stitched
behind the testis

Ligation of a varicocele

- A varicocele is a collection of swollen, distended veins around the testis (testicle). The swelling is caused by leaking valves in the testicular vein that allow blood to flow back to the scrotum on standing.

- Although occasionally present on both sides, varicoceles usually occur on the left side.

- In some men a varicocele causes testicular discomfort, that is often worse after prolonged standing or at the end of the day. Varicoceles also cause a small rise in temperature around the testis and this can affect the sperm and reduce a man's fertility.

- Ligation of a variocele is an operation to remove these veins. A small incision is made on the left side of the abdomen, through which a piece of testicular vein is removed. The two ends of the divided vein are tied carefully using self-dissolving stitches.

- The operation is usually performed as a day-case procedure under a light general anaesthetic.

- After the operation, you may feel some mild discomfort but this can be controlled with painkillers.

- Most patients who have reduced fertility because of a varicocele will benefit from this procedure.

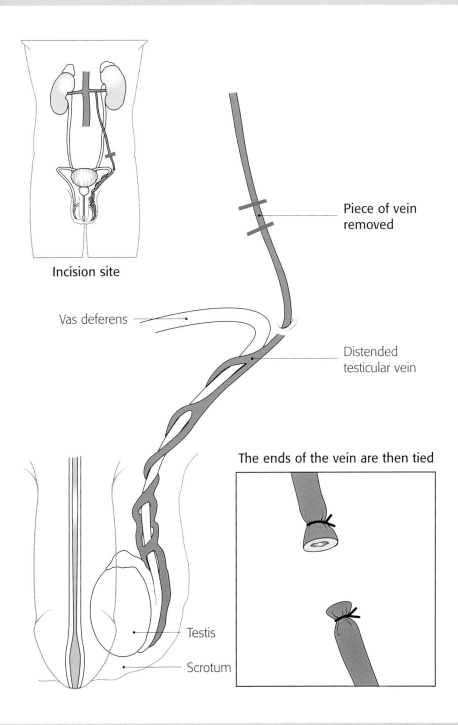

31

Incision site

Piece of vein removed

Vas deferens

Distended testicular vein

The ends of the vein are then tied

Testis

Scrotum

Radical orchidectomy

- Cancer of the testis (testicle) usually affects younger men (aged 20–40 years). It often develops as a painless firm swelling in one of the two testes and may be detected by self-examination or a feeling of heaviness in the scrotum.

- Testicular cancer is treated by complete removal of the testis on the affected side. This is called radical orchidectomy.

- The operation is performed under a general anaesthetic and takes about 30 minutes.

- You will feel some discomfort after the operation, but this can be controlled with painkillers.

- After the operation, you will need to attend the clinic for at least 5 years for body scans and regular blood tests to check that the tumour has not recurred elsewhere in your body.

- If the cancer has spread, further treatment with either chemotherapy, radiotherapy or more surgery to remove the affected lymph glands may be necessary.

- At a later date, some men prefer to have a silicone implant inserted into the scrotum for cosmetic reasons.

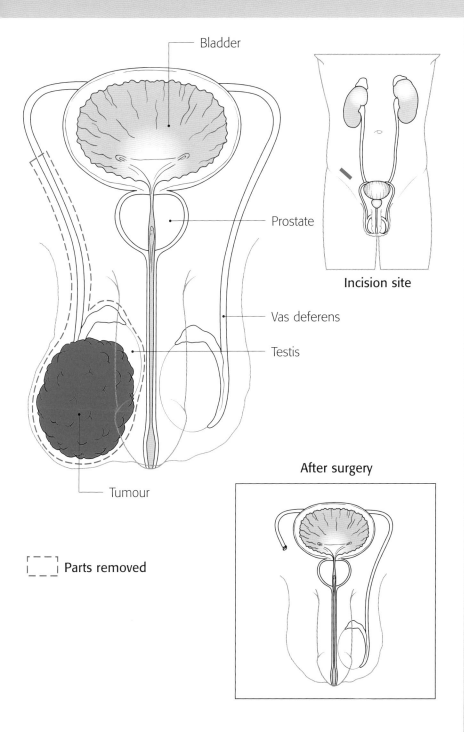

32

Bladder

Prostate

Vas deferens

Testis

Incision site

Tumour

Parts removed

After surgery

Implantation of a penile prosthesis

- The inability to achieve an erection sufficiently rigid for sexual intercourse is called erectile dysfunction or impotence. The most common physical cause is reduced blood flow to the penis as a result of hardening of the arteries associated with ageing. However, psychological problems are also common.

- A penile prosthesis is an artificial device inserted surgically into the penis, usually when other treatment options have failed. There are two basic types of prosthesis – semi-rigid and inflatable.

- The semi-rigid devices are flexible rubber rods that produce permanent semi-rigidity in the penis. Inflatable devices are more 'natural', in that they allow an erection to be produced as and when desired. The ability to deflate the device so that the penis becomes limp (flaccid) also makes concealment much easier.

- Implantation of a prosthesis is carried out under a general anaesthetic and takes about 1 hour. You will usually need to stay in hospital for 24–48 hours.

- There is a small risk of infection and so high doses of antibiotics will be given before, during and after surgery. Despite this, about 2 in every 100 prostheses have to be removed because of infection.

- Long-term results are generally good both for the patient and his partner, but some discomfort may last for 6–8 weeks. Occasionally, inflatable devices malfunction because of fluid leakage and may have to be replaced.

33

Semi-rigid prosthesis

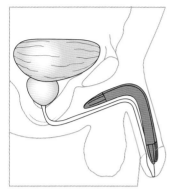

The prosthesis can be bent down, but true flaccidity is not possible

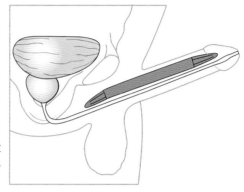

The prosthesis can be bent up to produce an erect penis

Inflatable prosthesis

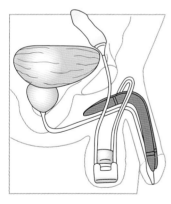

When deflated, the prosthesis is hidden

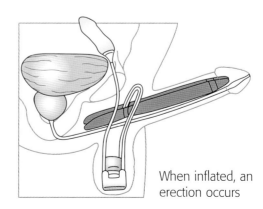

When inflated, an erection occurs

Mail order

This *Patient Pictures* book is one of a rapidly growing series. Current titles include:

- Bladder disorders
- Cardiology
- Erectile dysfunction
- Fertility
- Gastroenterology
- Genitourinary medicine
- Gynaecology (second edition)
- Gynaecological oncology
- HIV medicine
- Ophthalmology
- Prostatic diseases and their treatments (second edition)
- Respiratory diseases
- Rheumatology (second edition)

To be published:

- End-stage renal failure
- ENT
- Breast cancer

For further information about *Patient Pictures* titles or to order on-line, visit

www.patientpictures.com

Alternatively, simply contact:

Plymbridge Distributors Ltd, Estover Road, Plymouth PL6 7PY.

Tel: 01752 202301
Fax: 01752 202331
Email: orders@plymbridge.com

Health Press titles are also available at special discounts when purchased in bulk quantities. Please contact our Special Sales Department on:

Tel: +44 (0)1235 523233
Fax: +44 (0)1235 523238